KETO DIET FOR BEGINNERS

SYSTEMATIC GUIDE FOR KETOSIS
Lifestyle Easy start for WEIGHT LOSS

Legal & Disclaimer

The information contained in this book and its contents is not designed to replace or take the place of any form of medical or professional advice; and is not meant to replace the need for independent medical, financial, legal or other professional advice or services, as may be required. The content and information in this book has been provided for educational and entertainment purposes only.

The content and information contained in this book has been compiled from sources deemed reliable, and it is accurate to the best of the Author's knowledge, information and belief. However, the Author cannot guarantee its accuracy and validity and cannot be held liable for any errors and/or omissions. Further, changes are periodically made to this book as and when needed. Where appropriate and/or necessary, you must consult a professional (including but not limited to your doctor, attorney, financial advisor or such other professional advisor) before using any of the suggested remedies, techniques, or information in this book.

Upon using the contents and information contained in this book, you agree to hold harmless the Author from and against any damages, costs, and expenses, including any legal fees potentially resulting from the application of any of the information provided by this book. This disclaimer applies to any loss, damages or injury caused by the use and application, whether directly or indirectly, of any advice or information presented, whether for breach of contract, tort, negligence, personal injury, criminal intent, or under any other cause of action.

You agree to accept all risks of using the information presented inside this book.

You agree that by continuing to read this book, where appropriate and/or necessary, you shall consult a professional (including but not limited to your doctor, attorney, or financial advisor or such other advisor as needed) before using any of the suggested remedies, techniques, or information in this book.

Table of Contents

Introduction

It is to be noted, that you should ideally consult a physician before you start the Ketogenic diet. It is not advisable that you start a diet like a Ketogenic diet if you already have ailments related to the kidney or the heart. The first effect of having food low on carbs and high on fats is the fact that the kidney burns the fats instead of carbohydrates which end up putting pressure on the kidneys. That is why people with a pre-existing medical condition related to the kidney are especially advised to speak to a physician before they start a Ketogenic diet.

Below is a list of advantages that you can gain if you switch to a Ketogenic Diet plan.

1. It lets you control your eating habits and restrict your cravings for sugar and your fixation on food.
2. Ketone bodies are known to lower your appetite. This is especially useful for people who have an issue with food addiction.
3. Lowering many carbohydrates in your body also helps in reducing your blood pressure. If you are taking pressure medications, you might find yourself feeling weak because of being on a Ketogenic Diet plan. You may even be effective to reduce your pressure medications, after consulting your doctor.
4. Being on a Ketogenic Diet plan also helps you in bringing your cholesterol level down. Cholesterol comes from the presence of excess glucose in the diet and hence when in a Ketogenic diet you restrict the consumption of proteins and almost stop taking carbohydrates, the presence of excess glucose in your body is nullified. This helps in bringing the cholesterol levels in your body down.
5. Ketogenic diet forces you to consume more saturated fat, and as you do that, the amount of HDL Cholesterol (high-density lipoprotein cholesterol) in your body also increases. This is good because it improves the ratio of HDL to LDL cholesterol in your body. HDL cholesterol is a "good" cholesterol because it cruises through our bloodstream and removes harmful cholesterol from where it does not belong. If the HDL levels in your body are low, you are susceptible to heart diseases, but when it is high, like in the case of a body under Ketosis, the risks for heart diseases is considerably reduced.
6. A lot of people are startled to know that how useful a Ketogenic diet is for increasing your energy levels.
7. A Ketogenic diet almost removes any grain based food from your diet which many doctors think is a cause for stiffness and joint pain. Helping with stiffness and joint pain is one of the best side effects of being on a Ketogenic diet plan.
8. It has been noted that people who are on a Ketogenic diet seem to have greater clarity of thought than others. Some people attribute this to the fact that the brain is made up of more than 70% fat and the increase in fats in the diet enables it to function better. Others think that Ketogenic diet plans provide essential fatty acids and neurotransmitter functions to the brain which it is deprived off under normal diets.
9. The ketogenic diet is also known to help with reducing or normalizing your weight. Especially when combined with a technique of exercise called high-intensity interval

training, can increase the insulin sensitivity and in turn reduce the amount of fasting insulin and aid in reducing weight.

10. The ketogenic diet also helps in reducing heartburn issues by restricting the intake of grain-based food which is typically the reason a lot of people have heartburn issues.

11. The health of your teeth and gums are controlled by the pH levels in the mouth, which in turn is directly affected by the amount of sugar in the body.

12. Restricted intake of grain based food and low sugar also aids in relieving one of the digestions related problems as well. Once you have adjusted to a Ketogenic diet, you will find that there is a decrease in stomach pain, bloating, gas, etc.

13. When on a Ketogenic diet, the ketone bodies that are released to the body is also helpful in stabilizing neurotransmitters like dopamine and serotonin in the body. This helps in bettering your mood – probably one of the best side effects of a Ketogenic diet.

Thanks again for downloading this book, I hope you enjoy it!

Chapter 1: Ketosis

The "Plate" includes fruits, grains, and vegetables, and suggests that at least three-fifths of a person's caloric intake should be comprised of foods from these three categories. Incidentally, those categories are foods with high carbohydrate content. Fat is merely mentioned in the context of as oils, which are included as part of food "patterns," instead of being a major food group. Fats from non-aquatic animals, such as beef, pork, and poultry, are not included in the nutritional conversation at all.

However, many recent scientific studies have not only refuted that the exclusion of animal fats from the diet is a good idea. In fact, animal fat is not only an essential component of the human diet, but should be recognized as a major portion of human nutrition, especially when a person is striving to lose weight, and get healthier.

Ketosis

The human body was designed to use fat for energy, and when mostly fat is used for energy, it stores only minimum levels of fat. This results in a lean body, as nature originally designed it because excessive fat stores are not left inside muscle tissue, "padding" the body. If one goes on a high-fat diet, and the body is starved of carbohydrates, it will burn fat instead of storing it, and during the metabolic process, it produces "ketones." A high-carbohydrate diet, on the other hand, is more likely to result in weight gain because the body can quickly store carbs that are not used for energy and convert it to fat.

Ketones are molecules that are made in the liver from fatty acids and are generated from the breakdown of fats. Ketones are formed almost as a defensive action by the body: when the body "senses" that there is not enough sugar or glucose to provide for the body's energy needs, it immediately creates an alternative fuel source.

When dietary carbohydrates are suddenly taken away from the diet, more fatty acids are released from fat cells, which leads to fat being metabolized in our lives. This increased burning of fatty acids in the liver eventually causes ketone bodies to be produced and induces ketosis, a new metabolic state. Other hormones are likewise affected, and these help transfer the use of this new fuel, instead of carbohydrates, to body tissues. The majority of calories burned by the human body for energy will now come from this fat breakdown.

In short, ketosis is the process where your body burns fat instead of carbohydrates. When the burned fat comes from fat stores, then your body will be leaner, and the chances of having diseases associated with fat and sugar storage will be minimized, or even eliminated.

Getting to a state of ketosis requires ingesting less than 50 grams of carbohydrates per day, so having a fast counter booklet or app on your phone is the best way to start and continue the diet, to measure carbohydrate intake accurately.

Ketosis Mistakes and Misconceptions

It is useful to know what people, even health professionals, say that might end up scaring you off the Ketogenic diet. There are so many myths and misconceptions that have surrounded, and clouded, ketosis and the Ketogenic diet.

Ketosis Myths and Misconceptions

1. Carbohydrates are an essential nutrient for good health.

The truth: You can get nutrition and energy from protein and fat.

2. Eating a low-carbohydrate diet can lead to vitamin deficiencies, especially Vitamin C, which comes from carbohydrate-rich sugary fruits and vegetables.

The truth: You can still get vitamins and minerals from some fruits and other food sources

3. Ketogenic diets make your body to go into a state of ketosis, which is dangerous.

The truth: Natural ketosis is not harmful to your body. There may be some discomfort at first especially if you're used to a high-carb diet, but it's safe. The misconception is usually brought by lack of understanding of ketosis. Many people mistake ketosis for ketoacidosis, which is an entirely different condition.

4. Your kidneys will sustain damage from the high-protein consumption.

The truth: With a balanced diet, you should not worry about this at all.

5. A high-fat diet will lead to osteoporosis because it will cause the body to excrete calcium.

The truth: You can get calcium from sources other than dairies such as seafood and oysters, beans, and bone broth. You can even get it from dark, leafy greens such as kale and broccoli.

6. Eating fat makes you fat.

The truth: Dietary fat has little to do with body fat. You don't get fat just by eating fat. You become fat when your calorie intake is way higher than your calorie usage

7. The ketogenic diet leaves out carbohydrates completely.

The truth: You can have up to 50 grams of carbs every day.

8. Cholesterol from animal fat causes heart disease.

The truth: There is good cholesterol and bad cholesterol. Good cholesterol even reduces your chances of getting certain heart diseases! The ketogenic diet includes food that contains good cholesterol.

Ketosis, of course, means making fat, and to a lesser extent, proteins, a bigger part of the diet. This means relegating carbohydrates to a very minimum intake.

Common Mistakes On Going On The Ketogenic Diet
Because the ketogenic diet is a radical departure from what most people are used to, it is easy to make mistakes. The following are the most common mistakes that can eradicate the benefits of the ketogenic diet, and may even cause harm to your body:

1. To gain the maximum benefits from the diet, you have to be in a state of ketosis for at least two weeks - You CANNOT deviate from this, or you will need to start from zero again and allow dangerous carbohydrates to assault your system, and create even more fat.
2. Eating too much-processed fats and proteins - This is especially true for boxed or TV dinners. While they may have a lot of fat content, there are usually a lot of

hidden sugars, and worse, artificial chemicals that can derail your progress. Just because a boxed or frozen meal is high-fat does not necessarily mean is advantageous for someone who is on a ketogenic diet.

3. Eating more protein as opposed to fat - Fat will be your main source of energy, and eating excess protein can be harmful because some of it is converted to sugar.

4. Being afraid of fat - In the dietary world, fat is the friend, and we need to forget all the misconceptions about it.

5. Not getting enough water - Water is the most important element of any diet, and it sometimes helps to give the body a feeling of "fullness."

Chapter 2: What's Good About It For You

Low-carb diets including ketogenic diets have been under a lot of flak for a long time. Many people, unknowingly, were of the belief that high-fat content foods carry the risk of increasing cholesterol in the body.

However, for some time now, there have been multiple studies on ketogenic diets, and the results have been very, very promising. Ketogenic diets not only help in reshaping your body into an automatic weight loss machine, but they also have the capability to reduce metabolic syndrome related risks.

This chapter is dedicated to giving you some amazing benefits of ketogenic diets so that you find ample inspiration to get started on this wonderful journey that has the power to change your life for the better.

Benefits of Ketogenic Diets for Weight Loss

- Enhanced weight loss – Reducing carbs is the most effective way to lose weight. This has been the go-to way since the late 1800s for people to trim and drop pounds. There have been several randomized, controlled clinical trials on the turn of the century that showed people on low-carb diets lose more weight than those on a low-fat diet with the calorie intake being the same.

By preventing the accumulation of sugars in the body, ketogenic diets drive down insulin production. This compels our body to use up fat stored all around. Even when you are sleeping, the body will be burning fat for its needs! The fat that is being burned is not just the fat you ate but also stored body fat.

However, it is necessary to stick to the ketogenic diet that you started with unfailingly. Slowly but surely, you will see the positive effects on your weight.

- It helps you manage your hunger better – The ability to manage and control your hunger is extremely empowering. Hunger is, perhaps, the worst nightmare for anyone going on a diet. It also is the primary reason for people to give up their attempts halfway. Ketogenic diets, on the other hand, reduce hunger and food cravings as they keep you feeling full and satiated.

Fat is a very satisfying and filling nutrient, and ketone bodies reduce appetite so that you will feel far less hunger than before. In fact, there are times when you might just forget to eat! This is the most exciting part of a ketogenic diet. You are motivated to continue your efforts as you are not struggling with hunger pangs.

Counting calories is likely not going to be very helpful when your body is screaming out for food. On the ketogenic diet, you will feel less hungry, and your improved cognitive function will also allow you to judge better the amount of food your system needs.

- It enables effortless maintenance of optimal weight – Imagine your body being keto adapted and it is chugging along as an efficient fat burning machine. The value of effort that you put into maintaining or reduce your weight to hit your optimal range would be reduced just because your body is on the fat burning side this time! It is not busy storing up excess fats that your system doesn't use when there is excess glucose.

Exercising to keep fit, becomes that, and not a dreaded task just to burn off fats and calories to keep the inches off. Nutritional ketosis will open this door of letting you lose and maintain your weight effortlessly!

- It uses stored body fat as fuel – Yes you heard this before, and it won't be the last time you hear this, being keto adapted brings about a state where your body recognizes your body fats as a viable source of energy and proceeds to utilize it, thereby generating the ketone bodies for fuel. However, besides stressing the fact that your body fats are being burned while being in ketosis, getting your system to recognize those same fats as fuel also enables you to go on intermittent fasting much easier and quicker.

It is not the purpose of this book to expound the merits of going on intermittent fasting, but to reinforce that with your body's fats as a fuel source, should you wish to go on a fast, it would be much easier and the experience better.

- It enables faster and better recovery from exercise – On the route to losing weight, exercise would probably be one of the tools that can help. Now, it stands to reason that if exercise were to be helpful for weight loss and our overall health, wouldn't it be better if we were able to recover from those aching muscles and strains on a faster note than what we were used to?

One of the main known causes for those aches and rawness after a workout is essentially your body's systemic inflammation. That, in turn, has been linked causally to the presence of free radicals formed due to high amounts of sugar intake. On a low-carb high fat ketogenic diet, your body's systemic inflammation will go down as a result of lesser carbs and therefore lower glucose levels

This will not be the end where we talk about inflammation, but it suffices at this juncture to say that a lowered state of inflammation encourages body recovery after exercising and working out, and that is good news for most athletes and majority of the people who are keen on serious weight loss.

- It reduces and regulates the levels of insulin – Insulin is needed by our bodies to facilitate the usage of glucose or blood sugar. The insulin acts as a sort of messenger between the glucose and our body's cells, telling the cells to essentially open up and start using glucose as an energy source.

On a higher carb diet, our body would essentially be subjected to spikes of insulin every time our blood sugar levels spike due to the need to process it. That sugar has got to go somewhere!

Nutritional ketosis facilitates the reduction of insulin levels purely because your body has lowered levels of blood sugar through lesser consumption of carbs. The insulin spikes are also taken care of when your body switches over to ketones as the primary source of fuel.

Benefits of Ketogenic Diets for Health

- Improved cholesterol markers – Cholesterol markers like triglycerides, HDL was otherwise known as the good cholesterol, are known to react positively to the ketogenic diet. The LDL, generally known as the villain of the cholesterol panel, usually goes down in most cases regarding concentration while the LDL particle size, where the small dense sizes belong to the category of culprits that push up heart attack risks, normally increase in size to the larger, fluffy kind.

We must note that to get your triglycerides levels down, your HDL numbers up and be on your way to having those larger, fluffy LDL particles swimming in your bloodstream, we should be consuming not only a low-carb high-fat diet, but we must also note the facts which we are taking in. Saturated fats such as those found in fattier cuts of red meats or monounsaturated fats like those found in olive oil are the ones we should be concentrating on. Avoid any vegetable oils like palm, canola or soybean as much as possible for these contain polyunsaturated fats that are detrimental to health.

- Improved blood sugar readings – Again, a direct connection to increased consumption of sugar and carbs, blood sugar readings will show marked improvement when you switch to ketogenic diets. On top of that, the ketones which are brought about by the liver's conversion of fats also help out with chronic inflammation that is caused primarily by years of carb eating.

Ketones increase the response of the NRf2 pathway, which serves as a modulator for many genes involving inflammation and cell function. In general, the genes that encourage inflammation are reduced in response while the ones who serve an anti-inflammatory function are upregulated. This means that being on a ketogenic diet essentially reduces inflammation of the body. Besides aiding in muscular and workout recovery, the lowering of systemic inflammatory agents in the body also is a great help with cardiovascular diseases.

- Keto diets help greatly to treat metabolic syndrome – Metabolic syndrome refers to a medical condition that enhances risk to heart diseases and diabetes. The metabolic syndrome is, in reality, a collection of syndromes including:
  - ❖ High blood pressure
  - ❖ Abdominal obesity
  - ❖ Low HDL cholesterol levels
  - ❖ High triglycerides
  - ❖ High blood sugar levels

All five of the above symptoms can be managed and kept in check by switching to a ketogenic diet consisting of low carbs, moderate proteins, and high fat. Essentially, to reduce the risk of having heart disease, the key is to eat more healthy fats from whole and unprocessed foods!

- Ketogenic diets help with Epilepsy – This is returning to the literal roots of the initial usage of the ketogenic diet. Since the time of the ancients, the prescribed treatment for fits, which we now know as epileptic seizures, was to allow the patient to go on a fast or for the patients to not consume sugar or starches. Now we know of course that this route would set the body down the path of being converted to a fat burner and thereby produce ketones, which is the key ingredient for the effective treatment of epilepsy.

Documented usage began from the early 1900s where it was used as a go-to approach for epileptic seizures. You would have gathered from the early parts of this book that this form of treatment progressed well into the 1940s, where the inventions of antiepileptic medicines which offered fast relief of the symptoms, put this natural dietary approach onto the back burner.

Fortunately, the diet rediscovered some of its past popularity when Hollywood made a movie about it and right now, we have a healthy wave of adopters who are enjoying epilepsy-free lives without the side effects of medications. This proves that good things do last, yes sometimes they get buried and lost perhaps, but ultimately it will always come back if we look hard enough.

- Improving Fatty Liver Disease – Nonalcoholic fatty liver disease usually occurs in individuals who are struggling with obesity. It is potentially life threatening if it is allowed to go untreated and may result in liver failure.

You will need to know this, however, the fat that causes fatty liver disease doesn't come from any of the saturated or monounsaturated fats that you consume in your diet, but it is derived primarily from carbohydrates. The liver converts these carbohydrates into triglycerides which are then stored back into the liver as fats.

Being on the low-carb high fat diet reduces triglyceride levels because of ketosis, where fats in our body and also organs are the fuel for our system. With lowered triglycerides, the liver fat does not build up fat but instead regresses. In fact, some of the scarring on the liver due to fatty liver disease, known as fibrosis, have been known to improve.

- Ketogenic diets help fight many diseases - Ketogenic diets are known to have the potential to fight diseases such as polycystic ovary syndrome (PCOS), Alzheimer's, depression, traumatic brain injury, stroke and others that plague our present generation. There are many studies conducted by reputable institutions that have shown multiple promising results in this aspect. Cancer has also been one of the diseases which is receiving a notice with regards to the ketogenic diet due to the growing research on "starving" cancer cells.

The notion of starving cancer cells is not new, where it was brought up back in 1924 by German scientist Otto Warburg who proposed that the prime cause of cancer was derived from the fermentation of sugar within the body's cells.

The primary notion is to remove the sugar or glucose consumption, replace it with dietary fat and the cancer cells, starved of its usual fuel, will then die. It is this book's hope that more clinical trials and research can be done to further this hypothesis and who knows, we might just have a powerful deterrent for cancer.

Benefits of Ketogenic Diets for Lifestyle

- You will be more energized – Ketones are a more reliable and sustaining source of energy, and you will feel this energy surging through your body. Chronic fatigue symptoms that you had been experiencing till now will go away, and you will feel more energetic when you introduce keto diets into your lifestyle.

Due to the cut in reliance on energy from carbs, your body will be spared the "sugar rush" effect, where you get brief surges of energy followed by periods of fatigue. With ketones as your main energy source, your body will constantly be fueled due to the ever-present fat burning process going on, just like a lightbulb that remains lit consistently, without the flickers and intermittent outages.

- Your mood is enhanced, and there is increased clarity in thought – Both these improvements are credited to ketone bodies that are beneficial in stabilizing and controlling neurotransmitters such as dopamine and serotonin. The stabilization of these neurotransmitters helps you control your moods better and improve the clarity of thought.

Doctors who have tracked many of their patients on keto diets say that they have seen improved cognitive functions as well as reduced anxiety. The patients also tend to have better memory and seem to be able to enjoy and live life with lesser dependency on drugs and medications.

- Improved digestion – by shifting to a keto diet and reducing sugar and carb intake, you will experience improved digestion and your gut health will also see significant improvement. This is also associated with reduced sugar and grain consumption. The usual bloating and feelings of indigestion will tend to subside.
- Enjoy better sleep – With the adoption of the ketogenic diet, you will be more inclined to enjoy a good night's rest. Many ketos adapted practitioners report that after being in ketosis, they can sleep throughout the night like a baby, without sleep being interrupted in fits and being started awake. These improvements are linked to reduced glucose intake in the daily diet, which tends to facilitate a lower level of chronic inflammation in the system and thereby to allow the body to ease itself and remain easily in deeper rest.

Who Can Benefit from the Ketogenic Diet?

The answer to the above question is anyone who wants to get the benefits of such a diet. Anyone wanting to lose and maintain their body weight, anyone wanting to become more energetic and active, anyone who wants to manage difficult medical conditions like diabetes and more can feel free to get started on ketogenic diets.

However, there are some clear contraindications to keto diets. We are concerned with primary people who have a history of kidney, liver or gall bladder malfunction issues. The gall bladder is the store of digestive enzymes manufactured from the liver used to breakdown fat. Hence these two organs can be said to be fairly important for someone wanting to start off on the high fat based ketogenic diet. Here are some conditions that preempt a physician's approval before starting off on a keto diet:

- History of pancreatitis
- Impaired liver functioning
- Gall bladder related issues
- Impaired fat digestion
- Gastric bypass surgery
- History of kidney failure
- Pregnancy and lactation

While the previously mentioned above are a few conditions listed where it is encouraged that you see your physician before starting off on a keto diet, please feel free to talk to him or her anyway before embarking on your keto journey if you feel uncomfortable. Professional advice is always a good thing.

At the juncture, I would like to reiterate that ketogenic diets are not to be taken as mere diets but an embedded part of your new lifestyle. The effectiveness and success of ketogenic diets will be felt, experienced, and seen only when you find the discipline and fortitude to take the first step forward.

As you can see, ketogenic diets can help you get a lot of benefits, and it is those benefits which will keep you going when you take up this change in diet. Imagine being able to see the scales report back your loss of weight within a few weeks of being in ketosis, and being able to keep it there in the optimal range without fear of rebound. How about visiting your cardiologist after a sustained drive in ketosis and having him take you off medications for high blood pressure and other metabolic issues? These are not far-fetched notions and can be achieved with commitment.

A good ketogenic diet will help you get your energy from fats, a more sustainable energy source than carbohydrates. So, what are you waiting for? Read on, find some simple and delicious recipes in the coming chapters and start working on getting the benefits of a great ketogenic diet!

Ketogenic Diet Recipes

Breakfast Recipes

Low Carb, High Fat (LCHF) Coffee/Tea

Prep Time: 0 minutes; Cook Time: until the coffee/tea is brewed

Serving Size: 265 g; Serves: 1; Calories: 222

Total Fat: 29 g; Saturated Fat: 19.1 g; Trans Fat: 0 g

Protein: 0.4 g; Net Carbs: 0 g

Total Carbs: 0 g; Dietary Fiber: 0 g; Sugars: 0 g

Cholesterol: 31 mg; Sodium: 87 mg; Potassium: 120 mg

Vitamin A: 7%; Vitamin C: 0%; Calcium: 1%; Iron: 0%

Ingredients:

- 1 cup coffee/tea

Choice of fat source:

- 1 tablespoon coconut oil – 13.6 grams fat (11.1 grams saturated fat)
- 1 tablespoon unsalted butter – 11. 5 grams fat (7.3 grams saturated fat)
- 1 tablespoon cocoa butter – 14 grams fat (8 grams saturated fat)
- 1 tablespoon MCT oil – 14 grams fat (14 grams saturated fat)

Directions:

1. Brew the cup of tea or coffee.
2. Add 1 tablespoon coconut oil and 1 tablespoon unsalted butter, or your favorite blend of the fat source with coffee/tea, or blend as much fat source as you need to complete your ketogenic 65-75/20-30/5% fat/protein/carbs ketogenic ratio.
3. Mix the coffee/tea mixture well with a hand mixer until the coconut oil and the butter are well blended with the coffee/tea. The blend should be frothy.

Salted Caramel Pork Rind Cereal

These caramel pork rind cereals resemble salted caramel popcorn. The look alone will make your mouth water. If you are not a fan of cereal for breakfast, then enjoy them as a snack. These low carb, high fat cereals stray crunchy in the milk because of the caramel coating.

Prep Time: 5 minutes; Cook Time: 20 minutes

Serving Size: 250 g; Calories: 257; Serves: 2

Saturated Fat: 13.2 g; Total Fat: 23.7 g; Trans Fat: 0 g

Protein: 9.7 g; Net Carbs: 1.5 g

Total Carbs: 2.2 g; Dietary Fiber: 0.7 g; Sugars: 0 g

Cholesterol: 71 mg; Sodium: 413 mg; Potassium: 106 mg

Vitamin A: 17%; Vitamin C: 0%; Calcium: 24%; Iron: 2%

Ingredients:
- 1 cup unsweetened vanilla-flavored coconut milk, OR almond milk
- 0.063 pounds (1 ounce) pork rinds
- 1 tablespoon Swerve
- 1/4 teaspoon ground cinnamon
- 2 tablespoons butter
- 2 tablespoons heavy cream

Directions:
1. Measure 1-ounce pork rinds. Break them into smaller pieces that resemble cereal bits in sizes.
2. Put 2 tablespoons butter into a pan and melt over medium heat. While the butter is melting, put 2 tablespoons heavy cream and 1 tablespoon Erythritol in a ramekin and mix and then set aside.
3. Let the butter cook until it begins to bubble a bit, stirring if desired. You need to cook the butter until it's a little brown – this will give the rind color and a different profile to the caramel.
4. Once the butter is browned, remove the pan from the heat. Add the heavy cream mixture, continuously stir and then return to the heat. Continue stirring until the mixture is caramel.
5. Once the mixture is caramel and cooked down a bit, add the pork rinds. Stir and coat the pork rinds with the caramel sauce, makes sure each of the rinds is coated with the caramel.

6. Transfer the caramel-coated pork rinds onto a foil or a plate. If using foil, fold the edges to create a bowl.
7. Refrigerate the caramel-coated pork rinds for about 20 to 40 minutes or until the caramel coating is hardened.
8. Cook the chicken with the coconut oil in a frying pan until cooked through. Set aside.
9. When ready to serve, transfer a serving amount of pork rind cereal into a bowl. Add coconut/almond milk over the rinds. Enjoy with chicken.

Storing: Store the pork rind cereals in an airtight container and keep refrigerated for up to 3 days. You can double this recipe and have a batch of pork rind cereals ready. It's important that you choose the puffier and lighter pork rinds and not the very crunchy, hardened ones. Utz Pork Rinds have great texture. They will become crunchier as the caramel coating hardens.

On-the-Go Omelet Cups

These make-ahead cups are healthy and scrumptious. These cups are also kid-friendly. You can even bring these cups as your lunch.

Prep Time: 20 minutes; Cook Time: 20 minutes

Serving Size: 189 g; Serves: 4; Calories: 331

Total Fat: 28.1 g; Saturated Fat: 7.3 g; Trans Fat: 0 g

Protein: 16.9 g; Net Carbs: 3.2 g

Total Carbs: 4.6 g; Dietary Fiber: 1.4 g; Sugars: 2.1 g

Cholesterol: 381 mg; Sodium: 865 mg; Potassium: 360 mg

Vitamin A: 90%; Vitamin C: 32%; Calcium: 18%; Iron: 15%

Ingredients:
- 1 1/2 cups bell pepper, yellow, red, or green, diced
- 1 teaspoon salt
- 1/2 cup green onions, diced green and whites
- 1/4 cup whole milk
- 1/4 cups cheddar cheese, shredded
- 1/4 teaspoon ground pepper
- 2 cups baby spinach
- 2 slices bacon, chopped
- 4 tablespoons extra-virgin olive oil
- 9 eggs

Directions:
1. Preheat the oven to 350F.
2. Line a 14-15 muffin cups with silicone or paper muffin liners. If using paper liners, peel the wrapper before refrigerating or freezing.
3. Put the olive oil in a large-sized, cast-iron skillet and heat over medium-high heat. When the oil is hot, add the bacon, green onions, and bell pepper, and saute for 10 minutes or until the bacon tips begin to brown and the vegetables "sweat."
4. Combine the spinach to the skillet and cook for about 1-2 minutes or until wilted.
5. In a medium-sized bowl, beat the eggs together with the milk. Whisk in the cheddar cheese, pepper, and salt.
6. Spoon about one tablespoon of the bacon/veggie mixture into each muffin cup and then pour the egg mixture over the top of the fillings.

7. Bake in the preheated oven for 20 minutes or until the eggs are firm and the omelet cup tops spring back when touched.

Fluffy Coconut Pancakes

These nut-free and dairy-free pancakes are fluffy. Each serving is low in sugar and high in selenium.

Prep Time: 15 minutes; Cook Time: 5 minutes

Serving Size: 167 g; Serves: 4; Calories: 496

Total Fat: 43.1 g; Saturated Fat: 25.5 g; Trans Fat: 0 g

Protein: 23.6 g; Net Carbs: 3.8 g

Total Carbs: 5.7 g; Dietary Fiber: 1.9 g; Sugars: 2.6 g

Cholesterol: 287 mg; Sodium: 1007 mg; Potassium: 581 mg

Vitamin A: 7%; Calcium: 10%; Vitamin C: 3%; Iron: 22%

Ingredients:
- 6 eggs
- 3/4 cup coconut milk
- 2 tablespoons coconut oil, melted
- 1/2 cup coconut flour
- 1 teaspoon baking powder
- 1 pinch salt
- Coconut oil, for frying

Directions:
1. Separate the egg whites from the egg yolks. Sprinkle the egg whites with the salt and, using a hand mixer, whisk the egg whites until stiff peaks form. Set aside.
2. In a different bowl, whisk the egg yolks with the coconut milk and oil. Add the baking powder and the coconut flour. Mix until the mixture is a smooth batter.
3. Thoroughly fold the egg whites into the batter and let sit for 5 minutes.
4. Cook the pancakes in coconut oil for a few minutes each side over low to medium heat.

Freezing: If making ahead of time, let cool completely after cooking. Line a cookie sheet with parchment paper. Put the pancakes on the cookie sheet, placing the pancakes without touching each other. Cover with parchment paper and put another layer of pancakes. Place into the freezer and freeze until solid. When frozen, transfer to a gallon-sized freezer bag, label, and keep in the freezer. When ready to serve, reheat in the toaster, microwave, or oven.

Breakfast Stuffed Peppers

These stuffed peppers take a little effort to make, but they taste grand. With this make-ahead meal, you won't have to drag yourself in the morning to whip up something elaborate for breakfast.

Prep Time: 20 minutes; Cook Time: 35 minutes

Serving Size: 202 g; Serves: 4; Calories: 613

Saturated Fat: 27.2 g; Total Fat: 51.4 g; Trans Fat: 0 g

Protein: 31.3 g; Net Carbs: 6.2 g

Total Carbs: 7.8 g; Dietary Fiber: 1.6 g; Sugars: 4 g

Cholesterol: 235 mg; Sodium: 1573 mg; Potassium: 655 mg

Vitamin A: 48%; Vitamin C: 227%; Calcium: 5%; Iron: 14%

Ingredients:

- 2 bell peppers, your color of choice, choose peppers that are symmetrical with somewhat flat sides so that it's easier to balance them while baking
- 4 eggs
- 3/4 cup white mushrooms, sliced
- 1 cup broccoli, chopped
- 1/4 teaspoon cayenne pepper
- Salt and pepper, to taste
- 0.57 pounds (9.17 ounces) bacon, cooked crisp
- 5 3/4 tablespoons coconut oil

Directions:

1. Preheat the oven to 375F.
2. Dice your choice of vegetables.
3. In a medium-sized bowl, stir the eggs with the coconut oil, vegetables, cayenne pepper, pepper, and salt.
4. In a lengthwise manner, slice the peppers into halves. Remove the seeds and the core. Pour 1/4 of the egg mixture into each pepper half, adding more vegetables to a top and fill any space.
5. Carefully put the filled peppers on a baking sheet and cook in the preheated oven for about 35 minutes or until the eggs are cooked to desired doneness. Serve topped with hot sauce and with cooked bacon.

Storing: Let the stuffed peppers completely cool. Double wrap each pepper with plastic wrap, making sure that every part of the pepper is covered to avoid freezer burns. Put the wrapped peppers into a freezer bag, squeeze out excess air, and seal. Label and date the bag and freeze for up to 6 months.

Reheating: Transfer needed peppers in the fridge and let thaw overnight. Remove the plastic wrap and put the peppers in a safe oven container. Bake in a preheated 350F oven for about 15-20 minutes or until heated through.

Energy-Boosting Chocolate Granola

This breakfast treat is vegan and Paleo-friendly. It's an awesome energy-packed meal to start your day.

Prep Time: 10 minutes; Cook Time: 0 minutes

Serving Size: 120 g; Serves: 10; Calories: 231

Saturated Fat: 7.4 g; Total Fat: 17.1 g; Trans Fat: 0 g

Protein: 15.4 g; Net Carbs: 3.2 g

Total Carbs: 6.8 g; Dietary Fiber: 3.6 g; Sugars: 1.3 g

Cholesterol: 33 mg; Sodium: 261 mg; Potassium: 387 mg

Vitamin A: 0%; Vitamin C: 6%; Calcium: 3%; Iron: 14%

Ingredients:

- 1 1/2 cups sunflower seeds
- 1 cup dried cranberries
- 1 cup hazelnuts
- 1 teaspoon cinnamon
- 1 teaspoon salt
- 1 teaspoon vanilla extract
- 1/2 cup shredded coconut
- 1/2 cup unsweetened cocoa powder
- 2 tablespoons coconut oil
- 1 pound ground pork
- 2 tablespoons coconut oil, for cooking the pork

Directions:

1. Cook the ground pork with the coconut oil in a nonstick frying pan until browned. Remove from heat and set aside.
2. Put the sunflower seeds, cranberries, nuts, and coconut oil in a food processor or a blender and process/blend until the mixture is a rough paste.
3. Stir in the rest of the ingredients and store the mixture in a 2-liter Consol jar, Mason jar, or an airtight plastic container. Keep in the refrigerator until ready to serve.
4. Serve with a dollop of double cream plain yogurt.

Bacon and Mushrooms Breakfast Frittata

This make-ahead meal is greatly delicious; it's even kid-approved. Each serving is not only low in sugar, but it's also high in vitamin B6 and selenium.

Prep Time: 10 minutes; Cook Time: 20 minutes

Serving Size: 178 g; Serves: 4; Calories: 441

Total Fat: 37.8 g; Saturated Fat: 10 g; Trans Fat: 0 g

Protein: 22.7 g; Net Carbs: 4.7 g

Dietary Fiber: 0.9 g; Total Carbs: 5.7 g; Sugars: 2.8 g

Cholesterol: 290 mg; Sodium: 913 mg; Potassium: 422 mg

Vitamin A: 8%; Vitamin C: 5%; Calcium: 5%; Iron: 14%

Ingredients:
- 6 eggs
- 3 1/4 tablespoon olive oil, for frying
- 0.31 pounds (4.94 ounces) streaky bacon, sliced
- 0.22 pounds (3.53 ounces) mushrooms, sliced
- 1/2 cup cream
- 1 onion, chopped
- Garlic and chili butter, (about 1 tablespoon I can't believe it's not butter mixed with finely chopped garlic and chili)

Directions:
1) Put the olive oil in a heavy-bottomed pan set over medium heat. Add the onion and sauté until softened. Add the bacon and fry until almost crispy. Add the mushrooms and continue sautéing until cooked.
2) Add the garlic and chili butter and allow to melt into everything. Reduce the heat to low.
3) In a bowl, gently whisk the eggs with the cream and pour over the ingredients in the skillet.
4) Close the pan and let cook for 10 minutes or until the eggs are no longer runny and cooked well.

Storing: Using a spatula, loosen the frittata and transfer into an aluminum baking sheet. Let cool to room temperature, divide into 4 portions, individually plastic wrap, put in the freezable bag, and then freeze for 2-3 months.

Reheating: Transfer in the fridge and let thaw overnight. Serve at room temperature or reheat in a preheated 325-350F oven for about 1 minute.

Bacon, Spinach, and Feta Frittata

Although bacon is not ham, they are very close relatives that they will work with this version of Dr. Seuss' breakfast dish. Like Sam I Am who loves his green eggs and ham, you will love this grown-up recipe as well. The frittata is colored emerald by the spinach, creamy by the eggs, smoky by the bacon, and tangy by the feta cheese. The flavors blend perfectly well!

Prep Time: 20 minutes; Cook Time: 15 minutes

Serving Size: 233 g; Serves: 4; Calories: 451

Total Fat: 32.2 g; Saturated Fat: 12.1 g; Trans Fat: 0 g

Protein: 31.8 g; Net Carbs: 6.5 g

Total Carbs: 7.7 g; Dietary Fiber: 1.2 g; Sugars: 4.7 g

Cholesterol: 197 mg; Sodium: 851 mg; Potassium: 325 mg

Vitamin A: 31%; Vitamin C: 19%; Calcium: 20%; Iron: 15%

Ingredients:

- 7 eggs
- 0.42 pounds (6.70 ounces) bacon
- 1/8 teaspoons paprika
- 1/8 teaspoons black pepper
- 1/2 teaspoons salt
- 1/2 teaspoons garlic powder
- 1/2 cups milk
- 1/2 cups feta cheese, crumbled
- 1/2 cups onion, diced
- 1 turnip, peeled and sliced
- 1 1/2 cups spinach, chopped

Directions:

1. Cook bacon in a pan over medium low heat until crispy. When cooked, remove from pan and transfer to a paper towel-lined plate.
2. To the pan with bacon grease, add onion and sauté for about 3 minutes. Add in the spinach. Sauté for additional 2-3 minutes or until the onion is soft and the spinach is wilted. Transfer using a slotted spoon and transfer to a bowl.
3. In the remaining bacon grease, add the potatoes in a single layer. Fry until soft. Adjust heat to low.

4. In the bowl with spinach, add in the milk, eggs, garlic powder, paprika, salt, and pepper. Whisk together.
5. Crumble the bacon and add into the spinach-egg mix. Whisk. Pour over potatoes. Adjust heat to medium low. Cook without stirring until the eggs are almost set. Sprinkle crumbled feta over the frittata. Transfer to oven and broil for 2-3 minutes until eggs are set. And the cheese is melted.

Freezing: Allow the frittata to cool completely. Cut into six portions. Individually place in freezer bags. Freeze.

To serve: Transfer in the fridge and let thaw overnight. Serve at room temperature or reheat in a preheated 325-350F oven for about 1 minute.

Lunch Recipes

Avocado Turkey Bacon Salad

Ingredients:
For the dressing

1 tablespoon of olive oil

1 teaspoon of lemon juice

1 tablespoon organic apple cider vinegar

A little garlic (optional)

1 teaspoon of Dijon Mustard

Salt and pepper to taste

For the Salad

Extra virgin olive oil cooking spray

4 cherry tomatoes

100 grams of ham

2 hard-boiled eggs

30 grams of blue cheese

½ diced avocado

2 cups of coarsely chopped romaine lettuce

2 slices of turkey bacon

Directions:
1. For the Salad
2. Hard boil the eggs using the regular method, or a steamer.
3. Cut the ham into small cubes and then put them in an olive oil sprayed skillet for 3-5 minutes to heat.
4. Slice the eggs once boiled.
5. Place lettuce in an empty bowl then add in avocados, halved cherry tomatoes, turkey bacon, blue cheese, eggs, and ham, along with each other in rows.
6. Spread the dressing evenly over the top.

Nutrition Facts:
Calories 155

Cholesterol 400mg

Sodium 211mg

Potassium 132mg

Carbohydrates 2.1g

Dietary Fiber 0.1g

Sugars 1.55g

Protein 11.3g

Beef Scramble and Egg Whites

Ingredients:

1 lb extra lean ground beef

2 cups of regular or baby spinach

8 egg whites

½ cup of red peppers

4 small tomatoes

2 Italian tomatoes

Salt & black pepper to taste

Directions:

- Preheat an olive oil sprayed pan over medium heat then put the beef in the hot pan and let it break into large pieces.
- Divide the beef into smaller pieces while cooking and then put it in a bowl when it has cooked and turned golden brown. Set it aside.
- Beat the egg whites and pour them over the cooked meat.
- Sauté the spinach, tomatoes, red basil and peppers lightly then place them on top of the meat and serve while hot.

Nutrition Facts

Calories 167

Cholesterol 320mg

Sodium 121mg

Potassium 131mg

Carbohydrates 2g

Dietary Fiber 0.3g

Sugars 1.32g

Protein 11.3g

Chicken salad

Ingredients:

2 cups of baby spinach

½ or 1/3 large Avocado

½ chicken breast

1 tablespoon of Peri Peri Sauce

1 piece of low sodium bacon

Directions:

- Heat the pan over medium heat and cook the bacon until it has turned brown and crispy.
- Cut the chicken breast into equal parts while cooking. Put the chicken breast slices in the bacon fat and let them cook for 1 minute on one side then turn on the other side and fry for about five minutes. Before the five minutes are over, slice the avocado and bacon into small pieces.
- Put the avocado and spinach in a large bowl, and then add the peri sauce and bacon.

Nutrition Facts

Calories 178

Cholesterol 400mg

Sodium 157mg

Potassium 130.1mg

Carbohydrates 2g

Dietary Fiber 0g

Sugars 1.25g

Protein 12g

Ginger Beef

2 sirloin steaks cut in strips

1 small diced onion

1 tablespoon of olive oil

2 small diced tomatoes

1 crushed clove garlic

4 tablespoons of apple cider vinegar

1 teaspoon of ground ginger

Salt and pepper

Directions:

- Place oil in a large skillet. Once hot, put the steaks and brown them.
- Add the garlic, onion, and tomatoes when both sides have been properly cooked.
- Mix the ginger salt, pepper, and vinegar in a bowl then and add the mixture to the skillet.
- Cover the skillet, and maintain low heat. Let this simmer until all the liquids evaporate.

Nutrition Facts

Calories 168

Cholesterol 400mg

Sodium 202mg

Potassium 131mg

Carbohydrates 2g

Dietary Fiber 0.3g

Sugars 1.51g

Protein 11g

Stuffed Peppers

Preparation time: 10 minutes

Cooking time: 40 minutes

Servings: 4

Ingredients:

4 big banana peppers, tops cut off, seeds removed and cut into halves lengthwise

1 tablespoon ghee

Salt and black pepper to the taste

½ teaspoon herbs de Provence

1 pound sweet sausage, chopped

3 tablespoons yellow onions, chopped

Some marinara sauce

A drizzle of olive oil

Directions:

Season banana peppers with salt and pepper, drizzle the oil, rub well and bake in the oven at 350 degrees F for 20 minutes.

Meanwhile, heat up a pan over medium heat, add sausage pieces, stir and cook for 5 minutes.

Add onion, herbs de Provence, salt, pepper and ghee, stir well and cook for 5 minutes.

Take peppers out of the oven, fill them with the sausage mix, place them in an oven-proof dish, drizzle marinara sauce over them, introduce in the oven again and bake for 10 minutes more.

Serve hot.

Enjoy!

Nutrition:

calories 320, fat 8, fiber 4, carbs 3, protein 10

Low Carb Pizza

2 slices of low-carb bread

Cheese, 2 ounces per pita

3 tablespoons of tomato sauce

1 dash of garlic powder (optional)

1 dash of ground black pepper

1 dash of chili flakes (optional)

Optional

2 slices bacon

1 tablespoon of roasted red peppers

1 handful of spinach

½ cup of artichokes/olives/pesto

½ cup of pineapple/ avocado/mango/ Rooster Sauce

1 cup of pepperoni/prosciutto/salami/roast beef/ham

Directions:

- Preheat the oven to 450 degrees F.
- Spray the bread with cooking spray then put in the preheated oven for about two minutes until it hardens and then toast the crust.
- Mix the tomato sauce with the garlic powder, black pepper and chili flakes. When the bread is ready, remove from oven and add the sauce, and then the cheese.
- Spread with olive oil and then toast for another 2 minutes at a temperature of 450 degrees F until it crisps.
- Let it cook for another three-six minutes until the cheese melts completely.

Nutrition Facts

Calories 190

Cholesterol 400mg

Sodium 199mg

Potassium 128mg

Carbohydrates 2.1g

Dietary Fiber 0g

Sugars 1.51g

Protein 13g

Creamed Spinach

Ingredients:

10 ounces frozen chopped spinach

2 tablespoons cream cheese

3 tablespoons butter

Salt and pepper

Directions:

Remove the spinach from the freezer and put them in a microwaveable bowl then add 4 tablespoons of water, and then cover. Let these nuke for 8 minutes; check if they are done after the eight minutes- they are bound to be a little cold at the middle, so stir it up and set another 4 minutes in the microwave.

When done, pour into a sink strainer and drain it hard with a spoon. Transfer the spinach to a bowl then add the cream cheese and butter and stir until both melts and are fully consolidated and form a smooth sauce. Add salt and pepper to taste, and then divide into two plates.

Nutrition Facts
Calories 179

Cholesterol 400mg

Sodium 201mg

Potassium 130.1mg

Carbohydrates 2.1g

Dietary Fiber 0.1g

Sugars 1.4g

Protein 11g

Meatloaf

Ingredients:

½ cup of almond flour

2 cups of shredded and minced cheddar cheese

½ cup of shredded parmesan cheese

2 tablespoons of butter

8 ounces of softened cream cheese

5 minced garlic cloves

8 ounces of chopped white onion

2 large eggs

1 cup of chopped green pepper

1 tablespoon of thyme leaves

1 tablespoon of chopped fresh basil leaves

1 teaspoon of salt

¼ cup of minced parsley leaves

2 teaspoons of Dijon mustard

½ teaspoon of ground black pepper

¼ cup of heavy cream

2 tablespoons of barbecue sauce

2 lbs of ground beef

½ teaspoon of unflavored gelatin

1 lb of Italian sausage

Directions:

- Preheat the oven to 350 degrees.
- Oil a medium sized baking dish with butter and put aside. Whisk the Parmesan cheese and almond flour in a small bowl and place aside.
- Mix the cheddar cheese and softened cream cheese together in another bowl until a butter texture is formed. Place the butter in a medium skillet and melt it over medium

heat then add in garlic, onion, and pepper. Let this cook for about eight minutes until they soften. Set aside to cool and start preparing the remaining ingredients. Place the mixture in a food processor when it has cooled enough for a few seconds until the vegetables are minced.

- Take another small deep bowl, and blend in the eggs with salt, pepper, spices, BBQ sauce, mustard, and cream. Add gelatin on top and leave it for 5 minutes then mix the minced onion mixture and set it aside.
- Mix the sausage and beef.
- Put the meatloaf mixture back into the large mixing bowl and add the egg mixture and mix well. Add the almond mixture and mix well until the meat mixture does not stick.
- Cover a cookie sheet with wax paper and place the meat mixture to form a slab shape. Spread the slab with the cream cheese mixture. Fold the meat over the paper and roll it up starting at one end. Cover all the ends to protect the cheese mixture from spilling.
- Let this bake until browned at a temperature of 160 degrees F. Leave it for 5-10 minutes and then slice and serve.

Snacks and Side Dishes

Deviled Eggs

Ingredients:

6 large eggs

¼ teaspoon of French mustard

1 tablespoon of Hellman's mayonnaise

A few drops of hot sauce (optional)

1 teaspoon of paprika

1 teaspoon of cumin (optional)

1/2 teaspoon of cayenne pepper (optional)

Salt & pepper to taste

Parsley to garnish

Directions:

- Remove the yolk from the hard-boiled eggs.
- Using a fork, mash the yolk and add the other ingredients.
- Mix until everything blends in well to form a thick mixture.
- Fill the eggs with the mixture and sprinkle paprika on the top.

Nutrition Facts

Calories 177

Cholesterol 370mg

Sodium 210mg

Potassium 130mg

Carbohydrates 2g

Dietary Fiber 0.11g

Sugars 1.5g

Protein 13g

Egg Muffins

Ingredients:

6 Eggs

½ cup of Sliced Spinach

6 slices of nitrate free shaved turkey

Mozzarella Cheese

3 tablespoons Red Pepper

2 tablespoons finely chopped red onion

Fresh Basil (optional)

Salt & Pepper

Directions:

- Preheat the oven to 350 degrees F.
- Slice the red onions, basil, spinach, and red pepper and grate your mozzarella cheese.
- Spray a nonstick muffin tin with olive oil spray; gently drop the piece of turkey in one of the cups and let it rest at the bottom and the sides and expand the cup.
- Break an egg and pour it into the cup with the turkey.
- Add a little of the sliced red onion, spinach, red pepper, and cheese on the egg.
- Add fresh basil and sprinkle a little pepper and salt onto the egg.
- Put the muffin tin in the oven and bake until the eggs are set. If you want the eggs with a runny yolk, then ten minutes should be enough, but a harder one needs at least 15 minutes.

Nutrition Facts

Calories 169

Cholesterol 400mg

Sodium 200mg

Potassium 135.1mg

Carbohydrates 2g

Dietary Fiber 0g

Sugars 1.5g

Protein 13g

Stuffed Mushrooms

Ingredients:

1 lb mushrooms

½ cup chicken broth

8 ounces Boursin cheese

Paprika to garnish

Directions:

- Preheat, the oven to 350 degrees F., Remove the stems from the mushrooms and reserve them for another use.
- Fill all the mushrooms with Boursin, and place them in a baking pan.
- Pour some chicken broth around the mushrooms to fill the bottom of the pan.
- Spread lightly with paprika.
- Bake for 30 to 40 minutes and serve hot.

Nutrition Facts
Calories 155

Cholesterol 390mg

Sodium 154mg

Potassium 121mg

Carbohydrates 2g

Dietary Fiber 0g

Sugars 1.25g

Protein 12.1g

Dinner Recipes

Hot Chili Soup

Serves: 4

Calories- 396

Fat - 27.8g

Net Carbs- 5.8g

Protein- 28g

Ingredients
- 1 Tsp. Coriander Seeds
- 2 Tbsp. Olive Oil
- 2 Chili Peppers, Sliced
- 2 C. Chicken Broth
- 2 C. Water
- Salt And Pepper
- 1 Tsp. Turmeric
- ½ Tsp. Ground Cumin
- 4 Tbsp. Tomato Paste
- 16 Oz. Chicken Thighs
- 2 Tbsp. Butter
- 1 Avocado
- 2 Oz. Queso Fresco
- Cilantro
- ½ Lime, Juiced

Directions
1. Cut up the thighs and cook them in a greased pan. When they're done, set them aside to rest.
2. In two tablespoons of oil, heat up the coriander to release its flavor. Once it's fragrant, add the sliced chili to season your oil.
3. Add the broth and the water and let it come to a simmer. Season with the cumin, turmeric, and some salt and pepper.
4. Once it's simmering, add the tomato paste and the butter and stir until the butter has melted. Let the soup simmer for ten minutes.
5. Add the lime juice.
6. Place four ounces of thighs into bowls and spoon the soup over them. Garnish with the avocado and some queso fresco and cilantro.

Lunch Tacos

It's an easy and tasty lunch idea for all those who are on a Keto diet!

Preparation time: 10 minutes

Cooking time: 25 minutes

Servings: 3

Ingredients:

2 cups cheddar cheese, grated

1 small avocado, pitted, peeled and chopped

1 cup favorite taco meat, cooked

2 teaspoons sriracha sauce

¼ cup tomatoes, chopped

Cooking spray

Salt and black pepper to the taste

Directions:

- Spray some cooking oil on a lined baking dish.
- Spread cheddar cheese on the baking sheet, introduce in the oven at 400 degrees F and bake for 15 minutes.
- Spread taco meat over cheese and bake for 10 minutes more.
- Meanwhile, in a bowl, mix avocado with tomatoes, sriracha sauce, salt and pepper and stir.
- Spread this over taco and cheddar layers, leave tacos to cool down a bit, slice using a pizza slicer and serve for lunch.
- Enjoy!

Nutrition:

calories 400, fat 23, fiber 0, carbs 2, protein 37

Kung Pao Chicken

Serves: 3

Calories- 362

Fat- 27.4g

Net Carbs- 3.2g

Protein- 22.3g

Ingredients

- 2 Chicken Thighs, Bone In Skin On
- 1 Tsp. Ground Ginger
- Salt And Pepper
- ¼ C. Peanuts
- ½ Green Pepper
- 2 Spring Onions
- 4 Red Chilies
- 1 Tbsp. Soy Sauce
- 2 Tbsp. Chili Garlic Paste
- 2 Tsp. Rice Wine Vinegar
- 1 Tbsp. Homemade Ketchup
- 2 Tsp. Sesame Oil
- 10 Drops Liquid Stevia
- ½ Tsp. Maple Extract

Directions

- Chop the chicken into small pieces and season with the ginger, salt and pepper.
- Heat the pan over medium heat and once it's hot, add the chicken. Let the chicken cook until it's browned, around ten minutes.
- Chop and prepare the vegetables along with the peppers. Set it aside. Prepare the sauce by combining the soy sauce through the stevia together. Mix it well.
- Once the chicken has browned, stir it all together and allow it to cook a few more minutes. Add the peanuts and vegetables to the pan and cook another four minutes.
- Add the sauce and allow it to boil in order to let it reduce.

Grilled Short Ribs

Serves: 4

Calories- 417

Fat- 31.8g

Net Carbs-0.9g

Protein- 29.5g

Ingredients
- 6 Large Short Ribs
- ¼ C. Soy Sauce
- 2 Tbsp. Rice Vinegar
- 2 Tbsp. Fish Sauce
- 1 Tsp. Ground Ginger
- ½ Tsp. Onion Powder
- ½ Tsp, Minced Garlic
- ½ Tsp. Red Pepper Flakes
- ½ Tsp. Sesame Seed
- ¼ Tsp. Cardamom
- 1 Tbsp. Salt

Directions
1. Mix the soy sauce through the fish sauce together in a bag and then add the ribs. Marinate in the refrigerator for an hour.
2. Mix the spices and empty the ribs from the marinade. Evenly coat the ribs with the spices.
3. Heat the grill and grill the ribs for five minutes on either side.

Asian Pork Chops

Serves: 2

Calories- 272

Fat-9.5g

Net Carbs- 34g

Protein- 6g

Ingredients
- 4 Boneless Pork Chops
- 1 Star Anise
- 1 Stalk Lemongrass
- 4 Garlic Cloves, Halved
- 1 Tbsp. Fish Sauce
- ½Tbsp. Homemade Ketchup
- 1 Tbsp. Almond Flour
- 1½Tsp. Soy Sauce
- ½Tbsp. Chili Paste
- 1 Tsp. Sesame Oil
- ½Tsp. Peppercorns
- ½Tsp. Five Spice

Directions
1. Put the pork on a flat surface and pound it until it's half an inch thick.
2. Halve the garlic cloves and set them aside.
3. Grind the star anise with the peppercorns into a fine powder.
4. Add the garlic and lemongrass and blend until it makes a puree. Add the fish sauce, sesame oil, soy sauce, and the five spice powder and mix it well.
5. Put the chops into the tray and add the marinade. Turn it to coat and leave at room temperature for one to two hours.
6. Heat a pan on high and coat the pork with the almond flour.
7. Add the chops to your pan and sear them on either side, turning them once. It should be two minutes per side.
8. Transfer them to a cutting board and cut them into several strips.
9. Stir the chili paste and ketchup together as a sauce and serve.

Bacon Meatloaf

Serves: 6

Calories- 450

Fat- 33g

Net Carbs- 34.5g

Protein- 3.5g

Ingredients
- 1 Lb. Ground Beef
- 18 Bacon Slices
- 1 C. Almond Meal
- 1 C. Cheddar Cheese
- ½C. Mushrooms, Diced
- 1 Shallot, Diced
- 1 Egg
- 2 Tsp. Thyme
- 1 Tbsp. Salt
- 1 Tsp. Mustard Powder
- ½Tsp. Worcestershire Sauce
- ½Tsp. Pepper

Directions
1. Weave the bacon together as if you were making a lattice top pie.
2. Put the bread pan upside down on the bacon wave and flip it into the pan.
3. Mix the other ingredients together and try to keep it chunky rather than smooth. Layer the meat, add the cheese, and then add more meat.
4. Pull the edges of the bacon over the meatloaf and add another strip down the middle to make it look nice. Push down to make sure it's formed properly in the pan.
5. Cover it with foil and refrigerate it for half an hour.
6. Preheat your oven to 300 degrees.
7. Remove the meatloaf from the refrigerator and put the grill on top of the pan. Flip the loaf out of the pan.
8. Bake for an hour in the oven.
9. Turn the oven up to 350 degrees and cook another ten minutes or until the meatloaf is 160 degrees in the center.
10. Let it rest another ten minutes before you cut it and serve.

Fennel and Chicken Salad

Try each day a different lunch salad! Today, we suggest you try this fennel and chicken delight!

Preparation time: 10 minutes

Cooking time: 0 minutes

Servings: 4

Ingredients:

- 3 chicken breasts, boneless, skinless, cooked and chopped
- 2 tablespoons walnut oil
- ¼ cup walnuts, toasted and chopped
- 1 and ½ cup fennel, chopped
- 2 tablespoons lemon juice
- ¼ cup mayonnaise
- 2 tablespoons fennel fronds, chopped
- Salt and black pepper to the taste
- A pinch of cayenne pepper

Directions:

1. In a bowl, mix fennel with chicken and walnuts and stir.
2. In another bowl, mix mayo with salt, pepper, fennel fronds, walnut oil, lemon juice, cayenne and garlic and stir well.
3. Pour this over chicken and fennel mix, toss to coat well and keep in the fridge until you serve.

Enjoy!

Nutrition:
calories 200, fat 10, fiber 1, carbs 3, protein 7

Asian Pork and Shrimp

Serves: 19

Calories- 91

Fat- 4.7g

Net Carbs- 1.5g

Protein- 9.9g

Ingredients
- 1 Lb. Shrimp
- 1 Lb. Ground Pork
- 3 Green Bell Peppers
- 2 Red Bell Peppers
- 4 Green Onions
- 1 Egg
- 1 Tbsp. Soy Sauce
- 1 Tbsp. Sesame Oil
- 1 Tbsp. Minced Garlic
- 1 Tsp. Five Spice
- 2 Tsp. Fish Sauce
- 1 Tsp. Rice Vinegar
- ½ Tsp. Pepper
- ¼ Tsp. Salt

Directions
1. Prepare the shrimp and cut it into thirds. Make sure it's dry.
2. Chop the spring onions.
3. Add the pork, shrimp, spices, onions, fish sauce, egg, and oil to a bag. Mix it well.
4. Remove the air from the bag and roll it into a log. Marinate it for three hours.
5. Preheat your oven to 375 degrees.
6. Chop the peppers into quarters.
7. Spoon the bag mix into the pepper quarters and bake it for thirty-five minutes.
8. Turn the tray and bake anther five minutes.
9. Remove it from the oven and allow it to cool for five minutes before serving.

Conclusion

Thank you again for downloading this book!

I hope this book was able to help you to understand the ketogenic diet and know how to prepare various ketogenic recipes.

The Ketogenic Diet has existed in many variations over the years. In fact, it may have been the first diet humans have ever known. But the real question is: "Should I go for it?" Hopefully, by this point, the answer is a no-brainer.

If you are still deciding if this diet is worth your time, the only question you should answer is "What do I have to lose?".

Making big changes in life is never easy. In fact, most people delay making changes until they need to.

If you're 25 and in shape, make a change, so you're not 45 and overweight. If you're 45 and overweight, make a change, so you're not 65 and diabetic. If you're 65 and diabetic, make a change so that you're still alive and healthy at 85! It's never too early, or too late to take control of your health.

The Ketogenic Diet is becoming more and more popular because it works. It is not a fad, and it is not a trend. Studies keep coming out that show the tremendous benefits of being on a low-carb, high-fat diet.

Even good ideas take time before mainstream culture recognizes its benefits. Take a car, for example. It is something today that is universally considered a pretty good idea. However, when it first came out, people thought it was too smelly, too loud and too dangerous. A horse drawn carriage was considered to be a safer and more efficient mode of transportation!

There is a similar resistance to the idea of having a low carb diet. After all, fruits and vegetables are carbs! How can those be bad?

That is when scientific research comes into play. It shows people on a Ketogenic Diet diet burn more fat per hour, and has lower blood pressure. It also shows people that are on it have an increase in good cholesterol and a decrease in bad cholesterol. With more and more research coming out there will be a point where the benefits of the diet are undeniable. So it is better to start your journey on the road to greater health today.

Finally, if you enjoyed this book, then I'd like to ask you for a favor, would you be kind enough to leave a review for this book on Amazon? It'd be greatly appreciated!

Thank you and good luck!

Author's Afterthoughts

Thanks ever so much to each of my cherished readers for investing the time read this book!

I know you could have picked from many other books but you chose this one. So big thanks for downloading this book and reading all way to the end.

If you enjoyed this book or received value from it, I'd like to ask you for a favor. Please take a few minutes to post an honest and heartfelt review on Amazon.com Your support does make a difference and to benefit other people.

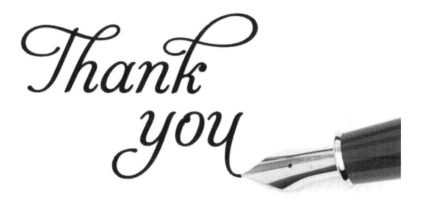

Made in the USA
San Bernardino, CA
06 May 2018